CW00521739

CONTENTS

THE COMPLETE HOMEOPATHY GUIDE   1

Copyright   2

Disclaimer   3

Fundamentals   4

Taking Your Cough Case   6

Deciding on Best Remedy   9

Administering Remedies   11

Dosage and Frequency   13

Potency   15

Sourcing & Storing Remedies   16

Cough Taking Sheet   17

Common Cough Remedies   19

Uncommon Cough Remedies   25

Croup Remedies   30

Sample Case 1   32

Sample Case 2   34

Sample Case 3   36

Conclusion   38

Glossary of Cough Remedy Names   40

About The Author   43

Books By This Author   45

THE COMPLETE HOMEOPATHY GUIDE

BY ANNE COLLINS

COPYRIGHT

DISCLAIMER

Any views, beliefs or opinions expressed or represented within this book are personal to the author, Anne Collins.

The content within this book, including text, graphics, images and other material are for informational purposes only. The content is not intended as a substitute for professional medical advice, diagnosis, guidance, or treatment. Always seek the advice of your doctor or other qualified health provider with any questions you may have regarding a medical condition. Never disregard professional medical advice or delay in seeking it because of something you have read in this book.

The author makes no representations as to the accuracy or completeness of any information in this book. The author will not be liable for any errors or omissions in this information nor for the availability of this information. The author will not be liable in any way for any losses, outcomes, injuries or damages from the display or use of this information.

FUNDAMENTALS

This book focuses on the use of homeopathic remedies for Coughs. It includes a wide range of remedies, both commonly used and less common, to treat acute coughs with home prescribing.

What Is An Acute Cough?

An acute cough is a short-term complaint which is self-limiting, not ongoing or chronic, and will clear itself anyway given time. It is not a deep-seated illness.

The remedies in this book are _not_ indicated for long-term coughs, asthma or any other respiratory complaint – in this instance, you should consult your homeopath and medical professional.

What Is Home Prescribing?

Also known as acute prescribing, these are the terms used for people selecting remedies for treating acute everyday complaints for themselves and their children or loved ones. This is done without the help of a homeopath and involves choosing remedies based on the presenting symptoms of an acute cough. Most home prescribers will have a stock of remedies in their home which they can go to whenever needed. If the chosen remedy is not in their stock, they can order it online, buy locally or borrow from a friend.

Benefits Of Using Homeopathy With Coughs

Homeopathy is a personal choice used by thousands of people throughout the world. It is easily available from homeopathic pharmacies, online shopping sites such as Amazon and some health food stores. It is easy to administer to all ages and is non-addictive and non-toxic. It can be used alongside other medications and treatments.

Many people use homeopathy in their homes because they are drawn to a more natural approach to their healthcare needs.

More Information On Home Prescribing With Homeopathy

Please check The Complete Homeopathy Guide series of books available on Amazon. These are books I have created from many years using and prescribing homeopathy for others.

TAKING YOUR COUGH CASE

When deciding on the best remedy for a cough, you need to take detailed notes on all the symptoms the person presents with.

These include the cough symptoms themselves and I've set out the best questions to ask below when gathering this precise information. But you should also include associated symptoms which are as a direct result of the cough. Examples of this could be energy levels, sleep, appetite, thirst and mood.

You do not include other symptoms the person may normally have. When deciding on a remedy for an acute cough, only take symptoms which are different to the "norm". For example, the person's norm is to be thirsty, but now they are thirstless – this is a difference and therefore should be noted.

The more detailed information you gather the easier it will be to select a good matching remedy.

Treat adults, children and babies the same way. If there are communication difficulties, as with babies, your own observations will be key.

Gathering Your Cough Symptoms

You should record the following information in relation to the actual cough –

1. Is cough dry or loose?

2. What does cough sound like? It might be raspy, barking, whistling, loud, dry, loose or something else.

3. Is the cough spasmodic (fits of coughing) or not?

4. When is cough at its worst? Some remedies have particular aggravation times – example would be Kali-carb aggravates between 2am and 4am.

5. What triggers the cough? What sets if off? Sometimes it can be random but very often there are definite triggers. The most common triggers are lying down, eating, laughing, cold air, changing rooms.

6. What helps the cough? Just like triggering causes, coughs can also be eased or improved in certain circumstances, such as drinking a hot drink, coughing up mucous, being in fresh air.

7. Any gagging, retching or vomiting with the cough?

8. If phlegm, how would you describe? What colour is it – clear, white, yellow, green? What consistency – thick, lumpy, stringy, watery? Any taste? Is it easy to cough up, or not?

9. Any pain with cough? Describe

10. Does changing position help or aggravate the cough?

11. Any other symptoms specific to the cough?

Gathering Associated Symptoms

Be aware that sometimes you might have a long list of symptoms whilst at other times you might only have one or two symptoms. This is fine as long as you have symptoms which are definitely a change to the "norm" of this individual.

When gathering symptoms verbally, always use the person's own words and descriptions. Don't make assumptions on what you think they might mean. Children are very good at describing their own symptoms.

What other symptoms are associated with this cough? These could be –

- Physical - discharge from nose, fever, headache, pale
- General – listless, hyper, better for warmth, worse for draught, better from cold drinks, worse when alone
- Emotional – irritable, sad, angry, weepy, bossy, want to be alone, clingy
- Observations – what do you see, hear, smell, feel? These are often key symptoms which should not be overlooked
- Anything else you feel is important

DECIDING ON
BEST REMEDY

If you are new to homeopathy, it can be daunting looking at the unusual remedy names and having to decide which is the best one for your case. Be assured that the more you use them the more familiar you will become to the point that you will choose remedies easily and effectively.

I have lots of free information on using homeopathy on my website www.annecollinsonline.com which is worth checking out if you are keen to use homeopathy in your home.

The general guidelines for deciding on best remedy are –

1. After you have gathered all your important information, look through the chapters of this book and select the remedy which best matches your individual symptoms.
2. Administer remedy as per Administration chapter within this book.
3. If you are unsure, pick the one that best matches what you are dealing with.
4. If you are torn between two similar remedies, you have a choice –
   a. Give one first for 3 doses, then change if first

       remedy has no impact.
   b. Alternate the remedies.
   c. Mix both remedies together if giving a liquid dose.
   d. Give both remedies together as a dry dose.
5. If you are dealing with a cough in more than one family member, it is important to note that different remedies will often be required. Homeopathy treats the individual, always.

ADMINISTERING REMEDIES

These are the general guidelines for administering remedies for acute coughs –

1. Take one pill initially.

2. This is called a dry dose as you are taking a pill directly into the mouth rather than a pill mixed with water.

3. If a positive response is obtained, there is no need to repeat the remedy unless this response begins to deteriorate again.

4. If the positive response begins to deteriorate, the remedy should be repeated. This step can be repeated until no deterioration occurs and the person is in an improved state.

5. If no response is obtained, repeat the remedy again. If still no response after 3 doses in total, it is time to look at a different remedy. Start again from Step 1.

6. You can take up to and including 6 doses per day (guideline only). It is ok to give more or less than this as long as a continued positive response occurs.

7. For babies and young children, 2 pills can be crushed

between spoons into powder consistency. This powder can be given direct or mixed on a plastic spoon of water. Please note that not all the powder needs to be given, a small amount will suffice.

An alternative way to administer remedies is in water. These are called liquid doses and can be used for all ages. Some people prefer to take remedies this way and find it easier, especially when administering to babies. The choice is yours.

Here's how to take a liquid dose –

1. Place 4 pills in a glass or bottle of water. Pills do not have to be dissolved before administering.

2. Take 1 teaspoonful to start.

3. Stir or shake x 5 times before each dose. This is known as 'plussing' a remedy and, by this action of stirring or shaking the remedy in water, it further invigorates the potency.

4. If a positive response is obtained, there is no need to repeat the remedy unless this response begins to deteriorate again.

5. If the positive response begins to deteriorate, the remedy should be repeated. This step can be repeated until no deterioration occurs and the person is in an improved state.

6. If no response is obtained, repeat the remedy again. If still no response after 3 doses in total, it is time to look at a different remedy. Start again from Step 1.

7. You can take up to and including 6 doses per day (guideline only). It is ok to give more or less than this as long as a continued positive response occurs.

DOSAGE AND FREQUENCY

The dosage depends on the severity of each individual case.

Frequent doses are often required for a cough which comes on suddenly and strongly and less frequent doses for a slower developing cough.

A more serious cough may require hourly doses until a positive response holds. Less serious coughs may only need 3 or 4 doses per day.

After you have given the remedy it is important to stop as soon as there is a <u>strong</u> positive response or improvement. If there is just a small improvement, continue giving the remedy but less often.

Prescribe up to 3 doses. If there is no improvement after this, look at a different remedy.

If the symptoms change, take the case again with the new symptoms (coughs can change). If the person is already under professional homeopathic treatment, and you are struggling to resolve the acute complaint, consult your homeopath for advice if possible.

Homeopathy is individual so you always have to follow the flow of what happens after you have prescribed your remedy. There are no 'definite' dosage rules. Just observe the remedy reaction and repeat remedy if symptoms deteriorate or there is only mild improvement.

POTENCY

The 30c potency is suitable for most acute coughs.

There are a variety of potencies you can use with homeopathic remedies. A homeopath will utilise all these varieties depending on each individual case. But for home prescribing purposes, the best potency to purchase is 30c.

Why 30c?

30c is potent enough to stimulate a reaction to the acute cough. But not potent enough to stimulate a deeper reaction on other levels.

SOURCING & STORING REMEDIES

There are lots of online homeopathic pharmacies throughout the world. See the glossary at the end of this book for the full remedy names you will need for ordering.

You can also source from a lot of the online shopping portals such as Amazon. Local health food stores often have a good range of remedies available, particularly 30c potency which is best for acute and home prescribing.

Store your remedies in a cool dark safe place. There are many urban myths to how you should store remedies which do not have to be followed.

COUGH TAKING SHEET

I have a free Cough Case Sheet which you can download and print as often as needed. Here's the link: https://annecollinsonline.com/wp-content/uploads/2023/03/Cough-Case-Sheet.pdf

If you prefer not to use the above link, here's some information which you should collect when taking a cough case.

Date:

Name:

Ailment:

Symptoms:

     1.

     2.

     3.

     4.

     5.

     6.

7.

REMEDY PRESCRIBED:

DOSAGE:

REMEDY REACTION:

COMMON COUGH
REMEDIES

These are the most common cough remedies used by home prescribers. Each remedy has a detailed description in relation to treating coughs. These remedies all have a large remedy picture but this book focuses solely on the cough elements.

Aconite

Dry hard loud barking cough. Comes on suddenly, usually at night around midnight. After exposure to cold or chill. Midnight is a big time for Aconite so coughs will often kick off just before or just after midnight. Feverish, thirsty dilated pupils (can look "shocked"). Anxious. Aconite is a good remedy for shock and fright so coughs which come on after an emotional shock or physical shock (cold wind to an exposed head). Good for early stages of a cough.

Ant-Tart

This is an easy remedy to spot. Cough is loud, rattling and loose. The breathing is also rattling. You can hear the rattling breathing from the chest. Lots of thick white phlegm. Tickle in larynx. Can yawn or gasp with the cough.

Arsenicum

Cough from an allergy or irritation in respiratory tract. Worse between midnight and 2am. Better for warmth and warm drinks. They will be cold, restless and very anxious. Worried about their health and what is going to happen. Thirsty for tiny sips of water (this is something you might observe).

Belladonna

Sudden onset. Face flushed red and usually an accompanying high fever. Dry violent cough. Headache. Chest sore from coughing. Moaning when they breathe. You'll feel the heat off them even before you touch them. Throat red and inflamed. Or feels hot and inflamed.

Bryonia

Slow onset. Dry stitching hacking and really painful cough. If dealing with a child, they will be crying at the thought of coughing, and will hold their chest in anticipation. Adults will be dreading the thought of having to cough because it is so painful. Worse for deep breath. Fits of coughing. Little of no phlegm. Very irritable picture – 'bear with a sore head'. Very thirsty. Will want to be left alone and keep really still as any movement whatsoever makes them feel a lot worse.

Calc Carb

Dry in the evening and night. Loose in the morning. Larynx feels irritated. Worse for damp weather and draughts.

Drosera

Dry cough. Violent spasmodic choking cough. Incessant. Deep and barking. Worse at night, particularly after lying down to go to sleep. Cough is suffocating, hard and deep. Tickle in throat sets off the cough. Spasms of coughs which often ends in gagging or even vomiting. This is a must-have remedy if you deal with dry night-time coughs.

Gelsemium

Cough with flu or virus. Sore chest with dry cough. Nose running. Chilly. Chest feels heavy. Feels weak and exhausted. Drowsy.

Hepar-Sulph

Rattly loose deep cough. Chesty & phlegmy cough. Phlegm is thick and yellow (same with mucous from nose). Feverish. Be aware the cough can also be dry and croupy too. Hates the draughts and the cold. Wants to be wrapped up warm. Extremely moody when sick! Irritable, impatient, critical.

Ignatia

Very emotional remedy. Cough which comes on after grief or an emotional upset. Dry hollow spasmodic cough. The more they cough, the worse it gets.

Ipecac

This cough sounds chesty or loose but usually no phlegm, or very little. Phlegm difficult to cough up. Choking irritating rattling cough. Ends in gagging or vomiting. May feel nauseous.

Kali-Bich

Rattling cough usually with sinus complaints. Lots of thick, stringy phlegm which can be hard to cough up. If there's anything going on with the sinus, think of this remedy.

Lachesis

Intense cough with sensation of constriction or something lodged in larynx. Feeling of lump in throat. Coughs all night disturbing sleep. Exhausted from cough. Cough much worse for talking. Worse for touching the outside of the throat or larynx, even pressure from clothes around throat. Jealous, suspicious, angry.

Lycopodium

Prone to dry tickly coughs. Feels like something is tickling the larynx. Head sore from coughing. Worse eating and evenings between 4 and 8pm. Better for warm drinks. Can be dictatorial within the home (opposite away from the home).

Nux Vomica

Cough after been excessively busy, stressed or overworked. Cough after over-indulgence. Cough worse mornings and particularly between 3 to 4am. Usually with a bursting headache. Better for keeping warm. Angry, quarrelsome, bossy.

Phosphorous

Dry hard tickly cough. Occasionally cough can be loose. Talking, laughing and changing air temperature can set off the cough. Tickling in throat and chest. Hoarseness. If there's any mucous from nose, it might be blood streaked. Good remedy for nosebleeds. Kids who get recurring coughs can do well on this. Colds that go straight to the chest.

Usually thirsty and prefers cold or ice-cold drinks. Asks for ice-cream. Anything cold! Usually worse in the evening, particularly at dusk. Chest can be painful during cough so person might hold the chest to cough. Lingering cough.

Pulsatilla

Very easy remedy to spot, no matter what is going on. Child will be extremely clingy and weepy. Adults will be emotional, crying and feeling very sorry for themselves. This can be a dry or chesty cough with yellow-green phlegm. Yellow-green mucous from nose. Post nasal drip. Phlegm is difficult to cough up and may taste unpleasant, usually happens in the morning. Always better for fresh air and worse for stuffy rooms. Thirstless.

Rhus Tox

Dry, irritated coughs. Painful cough. Worse after getting wet. Very restless, both physically and mentally. Will be up walking around at night with restlessness.

Rumex

Very tickly cough. Tickle especially of the larynx and upper respiratory tract. Usually starts off with a raw burning in larynx, then cough starts. Set off by change in air temperature from changing rooms, or opening the fridge or an outside door. Same when the air temperature drops during the night – so the person will cover their mouth to stop the coughing, or have their head under the blanket/duvet to breathe in the warm air. Incessant tickle in larynx.

Silica

Violent loose cough, worse lying down. Phlegm thick, yellowish-green and lumpy. Throat sore from coughing. Gags and trembles from cough. Feeling of hair being caught on back of tongue or larynx. Worse cold drinks and talking. Colds which settle in the chest. Very sensitive.

Spongia

Main remedy for Croup. But also for coughs that are really dry, barking, hollow and croupy sounding. Coughs can sound like a seal barking. Constant fits of coughing. Chest burning and sore. Voice hoarse and hollow. There can be a whistle to the breathing too. Aggravation time around midnight. There can be feeling that there's something stuck in the throat too. Voice might be hoarse. Cough is helped by eating or drinking. Much worse after lying down. If there is any mucous at all, then it is not likely to be Spongia (more than likely it has moved on to Hepar-sulph). Spongia is a very commonly needed cough remedy.

UNCOMMON COUGH REMEDIES

Even though these are less common, don't think that you won't use them at some stage. Some of these remedies are fantastic and once you get to know them you will start to use them more often.

Causticum

Cough hollow, dry and incessant. Tickling in throat. Cannot cough deep enough. Sore throat, larynx and chest. Voice hoarse. Very little phlegm which is difficult to cough up. Cough which disappears during the day but bad at night. Better for cold drinks. Often comes on after bad news, disappointment or feeling they were treated unfairly.

Chamomilla

Cough associated with teething in babies. The Chamomilla picture is angry and frustrated.

Coccus Cacti

Violent spasms of cough which produces clear ropey mucous

– either coughed up, or even vomited. The mucous might be hanging from the mouth. But the cough can be dry too. The airways feel raw. Worse mornings, particularly between 6 and 7am. Also 11.30pm at night. Worse becoming overheated, or in warm rooms. Much better for cold fresh air, or cold drinks / cold food.

Corallium

Dry cough. Spasms of coughing, suffocating cough. Can sound like a machine-gun. Violent spasms of cough. Face can turn purple with the coughing, usually ending with vomiting up stringy type mucous.

Cuprum

Spasms of suffocating or choking cough. Dry hollow sounding cough. Coughs themselves out of breath and will be trembling afterwards. Cough better for cold drinks. Nervous and restless.

Dulcamara

Cough when the weather turns cold but particularly damp. Worse for physical activity so if you are out playing sports or activities on a damp evening and this is setting off the cough, or brought it on initially, think Dulcamara. Throat tickles and feels raw.

Ferr-Phos

Short tickly irritating dry cough. Cough hard and dry, sore to cough. Spasms of cough, mostly at night. Good remedy when there is very little strong characteristic symptoms.

Hyoscyamus

Dry spasms of tickly cough caused by a dry itch in the larynx. Cough much worse on lying down at night and absent during the day. Cough exhausting with much sweat. Cannot sleep with cough and must sit up to cough. Tendency to curse and speak inappropriately. Silly behavior.

Hydrastis

Harsh cough. Loose with thick yellow/green stringy phlegm. Lots of gluey phlegm and mucous. Rattling cough with tickle in larynx. Nose also has thick yellowish-green mucous. Irritable and sensitive. Better for warmth and rest.

Kali-Carb

Dry hard choking cough. Worse between 2 and 4am. Painful cough. Incessant cough which wakes you up. Throat and larynx crawling and tickly. Better sitting up or bending forward to cough. Tendency to catch colds, which results in cough.

Mentha

Frequent coughs and colds. Dry cough that is purely caused by breathing in air through the larynx. The larynx and throat will be sore, even externally. Swallowing is painful, like there's a pin there. Voice husky. A big indication for this remedy is there are no major indications. So no real strong symptoms, just what is mentioned here.

Nat Sulph

Cough with ropey green phlegm. Lots of green phlegm. Must hold chest to cough as it is so sore. Throat feels raw and rough from cough. Chest fees tight. Much worse from damp weather. Aggravating time is 4am. Very irritable and does not want to speak or be spoken to.

Sambucus

Cough comes on around midnight. Cough attacks are sudden. Suffocating cough. Feels like cough is strangling. Wakes up suddenly feeling they can't catch a breath. Nose blocked so difficult to breathe out. May be sweating. Fretting with the cough.

Stannum

This is a deep cough which produces greenish phlegm. Cough can have a tinny sound. Phlegm may taste either salty or sickly sweet. Cough which starts from mucous caught in the throat or larynx. Cough starts from any movement, even laughing or walking. Person feels weak and exhausted. Anxious and sad about being ill.

Sticta

Cough which comes on after a cold or flu. The striking characteristic about Sticta is that the head cold dries up and within hours the cough starts. Dry, constant, hacking cough. Becomes exhausted with the cough. Worse at night and practically absent during the day. Person will be talkative.

Sulphur

Unresolved loose cough. Chest feels tight. Worse at night when lying down in bed which disturbs sleep. Worse for warmth and being overheated. Better for fresh air. Feels hot and feverish.

Headache which feels hot. Phlegm is yellowish-green and sticky and rattles in chest. Acts selfishly with explosive temper when told what to do.

CROUP REMEDIES

These are the main croup remedies. Spongia is the most common remedy for croup. Check the other chapters for more information on these remedies.

Aconite

Dry hard barking cough, comes on around midnight. Often accompanied with fever. First early stage of croup.

Hepar-Sulph

Loose croup cough. Yellow phlegm.

Phosphorous

Dry tickly cough. Hoarse. Thirsty.

Sambucus

Suffocating cough, phlegm difficult to cough up.

Spongia

Main remedy for croup. Comes on around midnight. Dry barking cough which often sounds like a seal.

SAMPLE CASE 1

Tom is age 9 and has a bit of a cough during the day but it gets much worse at night after he lies down and goes to sleep. Seems to kick off about 10pm. It gets bad then and he is having fits of cough, so much that he often retches after a spasm. The cough is dry with no phlegm and the cough just goes on and on for hours. He wakes up feeling pretty miserable and wants his mum or dad to stay with him.

What Are The Top Symptoms To Take Note Of?

Dry Cough

Worse after lying down at night

Incessant cough

Which Is Best Remedy?

Drosera 30

Suggested Dosage

Drosera 30c dry pill straight into his mouth. Every 30 minutes for 4 doses or until cough has eased or he goes back to sleep. Repeat during night if he wakes with cough. The next day, give 4 doses spread throughout the day.

SAMPLE CASE 2

Jane is age 7 and she has a chesty cough. She is coughing up phlegm which is yellow and thick. She wants to be wrapped up warm and you observe that she is a little sensitive and snappy. She also has mucous from the nose which is yellow.

What Are The Top Symptoms To Take Note Of?

Loose cough

Phlegm yellow

Phlegm thick

Nose mucous, yellow

Better for warmth

Which Is Best Remedy?

The two remedies that are indicated are Hepar-sulph and Hydrastis. But Jane is not overly irritable which suggests that Hydrastis is a better match.

Hydrastis 30c

Suggested Dosage

Hydrastis 30c liquid dose (or dry, according to personal preference). 4 doses per day until symptoms have responded positively and Jane is feeling better again.

SAMPLE CASE 3

Maggie is an adult and she can feel a cough starting one evening. She was out for a hill walk earlier in the day and had forgotten her hat. She knows that she has a sensitive head to the weather, particularly wind, which often triggers a cough or earache. Her throat is tickly and she is starting to cough. She feels warm and not very well. Her nose has also started to run and there is a tiny streak of red in it. She is craving water with lots of ice cubes.

What Are The Top Symptoms To Take Note Of?

Early stage cough

Cough after exposure to wind

Tickly throat

Nose mucous streaked red

Craving cold drinks

Which Is Best Remedy?

The two remedies that are indicated are Aconite and Phosphorous. Either remedy would be a good match in this situation, particularly as the cough has not progressed enough to present more established symptoms. I would prescribe Phosphorous first because of the cravings for cold drinks and the red-streaked mucous.

Phosphorous 30c

Suggested Dosage

Phosphorous 30c, two doses before bed. Repeat during night if cough wakes her. Also keep in mind Aconite, particularly if symptoms deteriorate rapidly around midnight.

CONCLUSION

If you are new to homeopathy don't be afraid to have a go and try some of these amazing remedies.

Have remedies in your home so you are ready to react if a cough presents. It is a good idea to go through the remedies listed in this book to see if any resonate with your own family trends. Then you can keep them in your first aid store. There is no need to buy a Remedy Kit unless you are fully sure you will use every remedy in the box. Very often people find that they gravitate towards particular remedies in the box then the rest are left unused. My recommendation is buy what you need and build your stock gradually. I have lots of blogs on my website www.annecollineonline.com with recommended remedy lists for building your stock.

Check out my other books within The Complete Homeopathy Guide series. They are all available on Amazon.

If you find that coughs become a recurring complaint for you or your loved one consider consulting with a professional homeopath. It is OK to treat the cough episode with home prescribing, but sometimes a deeper remedy is required.

Lastly, I'd like to thank you for buying this book and I hope you find it beneficial for your home prescribing. Don't let fear stop you selecting remedies, set your intention and have good reasons for selecting your chosen remedy.

Go forth and prescribe!

Anne xxx

GLOSSARY OF COUGH REMEDY NAMES

Abbreviation	Remedy Full Name
Acon	Aconite (Aconitum Napellus)
Ant-t	Ant Tart (Antimonium Tartaricum)
Ars	Arsenicum (Arsenicum Album)
Bell	Belladonna
Bry	Bryonia (Bryonia Alba)
Calc	Calc Carb (Calcarea Carbonica)
Caust	Causticum
Cham	Chamomilla (Chamomilla Vulgaris)
Coc-c	Coccus Cacti
Cor-r	Corallium (Corallium Rubrum)
Cupr	Cuprum (Cuprum Metallicum)
Dros	Drosera (Drosera Rotundifolia)
Dulc	Dulcamara
Ferr-p	Ferr-phos (Ferrum Phosphoricum)
Gels	Gelsemium (Gelsemium Sempervirens)
Hep	Hepar Sulph (Hepar Sulphuris Calcareum)
Hyos	Hyoscyamus (Hyoscyamus Niger)

Hydr	Hydrastis (Hydrastis Canadensis)
Ign	Ignatia (Ignatia Amara)
Ip	Ipecac (Ipecacuanha)
Kali-b	Kali-bich (Kali Bichromicum)
Kali-c	Kali-carb (Kali Carbonicum)
Lach	Lachesis (Lachesis Muta)
Lyc	Lycopodium (Lycopodium Clavatum)
Menth	Mentha (Mentha Piperita)
Nat-s	Nat Sulph (Natrum Sulphuricum)
Nux-v	Nux Vomica
Phos	Phosphorous
Puls	Pulsatilla (Pulsatilla Nigricans)
Rhus	Rhus Tox (Rhus Toxicodendron)
Rumx	Rumex (Rumex Crispus)
Samb	Sambucus (Sambucus Nigra)
Sil	Silica (Silica Terra)
Spon	Spongia (Spongia Tosta)
Stann	Stannum Metallicum
Sticta	Sticta Pulmonaria
Sulph	Sulphur

ABOUT THE AUTHOR

Anne Collins

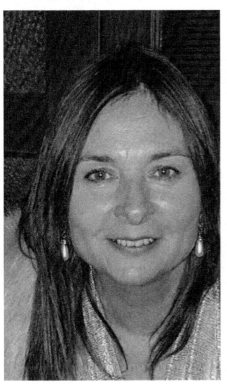

Anne Collins is an Irish Homeopath with 20+ years experience. She has worked with people around the world prescribing remedies for various complaints.

She is currently writing a full series of homeopathy books focused on making homeopathy accessible to all.

She has a busy blog with lots of free information on homeopathy.

BOOKS BY THIS AUTHOR

The Complete Homeopathy Guide - For Everyday Complaints

Easy to use homeopathy book which gives you the confidence and know-how to choose remedies wisely for your own and your family's acute everyday complaints.

The Complete Homeopathy Guide - For Baby & Toddler

Very user friendly and suitable for all levels. You will learn how to choose remedies, how to administer and how to dose. Included are the top remedies for specific ailments seen in this ae group such as colic, reflux, coughs, croup, teething, earaches, sore throats and much more.

Printed in Great Britain
by Amazon

40680572R00030